C.P. CUSON

HERBAL ANTIBIOTICS

The Essential Guide to Natural Herbal Remedies, Learn All The Natural Cures For Different Ailments Your Doctor Never Told You About

Descrierea CIP a Bibliotecii Naţionale a României
C.P. CUSON
    HERBAL ANTIBIOTICS. The Essential Guide to Natural
Herbal Remedies, Learn All The Natural Cures For Different
Ailments Your Doctor Never Told You About / C.P. Cuson. –
Bucharest: Editura My Ebook, 2020
    ISBN

C.P. CUSON

HERBAL ANTIBIOTICS

The Essential Guide to Natural Herbal Remedies, Learn All The Natural Cures For Different Ailments Your Doctor Never Told You About

My Ebook Publishing House
Bucharest, 2020

TABLE OF CONTENTS

CONVENTIONAL CURES
VS NATURAL HERBAL CURE

According to the American Medical Association Journal, over 100,000 Americans die in hospitals every year due to side effects from regularly prescribed medications. Throughout America, a huge amount of medication is prescribed on a daily basis. The medical community openly acknowledges that fact that it does not have any cure for several common diseases that affect people.

Most allopathic medicines have side effects that can range from mild to severe. The reason for this is that most of these chemicals have certain toxic properties. This is why there have been so many prescription drugs that got pulled from the market after enjoying several years of FDA approval.

The sad thing is that very few doctors nowadays bother to inform patients about possible side effects due to close and cozy relationships with the pharmaceutical industries.

Half of the truth is that pharmaceutical companies will only tell doctors as much as they want to and not reveal the complete picture. Therefore, the doctors are not completely to blame because they cannot warn patients against side effects of chemicals they are not aware of.

The trouble is that the business is so profitable is that these medicine manufacturers are more concerned with profits and FDA approval rather than the overall effect on the patients.

This is one reason why several doctors are now beginning to recommend complementary alternative treatments, like herbal therapies and medicines.

Here are some interesting facts:

- The totally amount of annual profits made by pharmaceutical companies through sale of drugs in the United States alone is over $100 billion
- More than 25% of all prescription drugs available contain plant derivatives
- More than 80,000 types of plants are used all over the world for medicinal purposes
- Over 75% of the global population depends on herbal remedies for regular treatment

There are several choices available for people who are looking for alternative remedies, including Acupuncture, Yoga, Qigong, Tai chi, Ayurveda, hydrotherapy, massage therapy, homeopathy, energy medicines, holistic approaches, and aromatherapy. In fact, the number of herbal remedies available for different ailments equals (if not exceeds) the number of regular drug treatments provided by pharmaceutical companies.

The point is that prevention always was and always will be better than any cure, mainstream or alternative. The advantage of herbal remedies is that they move an individual towards a lifestyle more geared toward prevention and cure in the early stages of any affliction.

Pharmaceutical drugs work only after the problem has development, they do not try to prevent problems because then the manufacturing companies would go into a loss.

This is where herbal remedies leave the mainstream drugs behind. This is also the reason why so many people are daily turning to herbal therapies.

Herbal remedies treat the cause of the disease and not the symptoms (like conventional drugs). Herbal remedies also have almost no side effects.

THE ALTERNATIVE CURE ADVANTAGE

Alternative medicine believes that natural health is a consequence of a variety of different sources coming together. Thus it chooses the best from various options available, in order to provide good health. It does so by building the strong points, preventing the weak ones, and generally dictating a lifestyle that is naturally healthy. Alternative medicine branches that promote natural good health include herbalism, natural hygiene, naturotherapy, and nutripathy. Nowadays it has become common to provide these, as complementary therapies to conventional methods of treatment. Terms like alternative medicine and natural health always seem to get associated with the Far East. It should be noted that most of the core concepts behind natural health are of European origin.

In the old age the only health care that was available to the common man was self care. While medical science existed in a very rudimentary state, it was by no means as prolific as it is today. Most of the "doctors" in that era were referred to as "folk healers" (people who heal other people) and their medical qualification was nothing more than a short apprenticeship under some sort of superior.

At the time of the Revolutionary War, practicing the art of medicinal healing was looked upon as a diversion, something to dabble in when you had time to spare. It was supposed to be something that an individual did when not doing a regular job. Folk remedies were handed down from one generation to the next. Men and women who had learned these remedies simply applied them to everyday life like their predecessors. In this way, matters like childbirth, injuries, and illness were taken care of.

Geographical distance and biological diversity naturally made these folk remedies different in different places. So, while the roots of such healing can be traced to Europe, once they had been adapted to the Americas, they were not so readily recognizable.

In 1830, Frances Wright and other reformers and activists started the Popular Health Movement. This was a period when advances in medical science were forcing contemporary doctors to think in terms that would have been sacrilegious to their elders. Frustrated by these new developments, proponents of the

Popular Health Movement sought to enforce the usage of older methods into the practice of modern medical professionals. While some good has resulted (in the long run and with the help of understanding provided by modern research), it has to be admitted that the Popular Health Movement also caused some medical blunders.

Some natural health concepts that arose as a result of the Popular Health Movement are: Hydrotherapy, Herbalism, Eclectic Medicine, and Natural Hygiene.

Thomsonianism is one of the earliest approaches to modern western herbalism and it was founded by Samuel Thompson around the year 1820.

The Association of Eclectic Physicians, an organization of herbals doctors, was found in Wooster Beech.

At its very height, eclecticism was practiced by over twenty thousand qualified doctors in the United States. By 1939, medical schools were being largely influenced by philanthropists, and when these schools failed to support eclecticism, it slowly died out.

Hydrotherapy was another branch of natural health and it concerned itself with the application of water to the human body. Though using only water as means of staying healthy might sound a bit silly, for that time period it was a good thing.

Hydrotherapy advocates were very vocal about the importance of personal habits such as diet, dress, clean water, fresh air, exercise, sunshine, and herbs. Personal hygiene as it is followed today was not always such an important issue. Hydrotherapy was conveying a very important message. Origins of hydrotherapy can be traced back to Europe in the Roman era when spas and hot mineral springs were a common way for people to cleanse their bodies.

The European system of hydrotherapy was first introduced to the United States in 1844 by the founder of Natural Hygiene, Dr. Joel Shew. Dr. Shew later on enhanced hydrotherapy by focusing on its other aspects like fresh air, lots of sunshine, a good diet plan, and an exercise routine. In 1853 he established the college of Hygieo Therapy.

The American Natural Hygiene Society was founded in 1948. Eventually, hydrotherapy had to give way to allopathy. This was largely brought about by the fact that the people supporting allopathy viewed hydrotherapy as a science of quacks because hydrotherapy was so closely associated with the female social activists of that era.

The core belief of natural health therapy is that all issues related to health, sickness, and healing can be overcome through simple means like prevention and a change in individual lifestyle. Natural health follows the oldest rule of medicine: prevention is better than cure. In view of this, natural health therapies are supposed to be totally in control of the individual and not the doctor or healer.

The "natural" in the term natural health literally refers to the physical world in which we live, or nature. This is but another way of saying that according to natural health therapy all disease and illness is nothing more than a natural reaction to some other natural action. It is important to remember that natural health does not have anything to do with faith or psychic healing which are supernatural concepts and hence,

By definition, not part of nature. This difference is also the biggest distinguishing factor between natural health therapies of European origin and Eastern alternative medicinal theories that often rely on belief systems such as spirituality, karma, ancestral forces, personal auras, or energy flows. None of these can be perceived by our normal senses and hence the Europe-born natural health theories do not subscribe to them.

Going even further, natural health does not concern itself with the origin of life, any religious beliefs, extra-dimensional worlds, magic, and new age mysticism.

All natural health says is that all health and sickness can be affected by simple natural therapies.

At its most basic level it can be said that natural health therapy refers to only one thing: biological factors of health, especially as they apply to everyday life in western society. In its early history, the natural health movement did show considerable interest in hydrotherapy and the relaxation it offered through the usage of spas, steam baths, and other water cures. The more modern additions to natural health that concern themselves with the body-mind connection and how that relates to stress and tension are influenced by eastern alternative medical theories.

Having said that, what natural health therapy finally implies is that the human body has complete capacity to heal itself from most forms of sickness (of course, a broken bone cannot be fixed by altering your lifestyle, it needs to be put in a cast), mostly through prevention. So as far as natural health thinking goes, all healing is basically self-healing and this is considered to be a basic property of all things alive.

Vitalism

It is to be observed that as early 400 B.C., Hippocrates (who is considered to be the father of medicine) had written that, "the natural healing force within us is the greatest force in getting well".

This is known as vitalism, also known as 'vis medicatrix naturae' (the inherent wisdom of the body).

To put it simply, whenever there is something wrong with the body the doctor will attempt something, for example: using antibiotics to kill the infection, perform surgery to remove a poisoned part or for amputation, put a broken bone into a cast, suture a flesh wound. All of these are part of the healing trade. The catch is that the body of patient has to actively respond to all this treatment otherwise it is wasted. Vitalism makes the body want to heal and get well. This is a well documented fact that people who deal with their physical problems confidently and cheerfully heal faster than others. The precise reason as to why this happens is not understood but the fact is still undeniable.

Holism

One explanation comes from the concept of Holism which says that the process of healing is a combined effort by the entire organism and cannot be achieved by any isolated part of that organism.

The Holism concept can be traced to the time of Paracelsus, 1439- 1541, who is credited with being the father of modern medicine.

When Paracelsus treated patients he refused to pay attention to only that part which was showing symptoms of disease. Instead, he tried to treat the whole body as one whole entity.

Holism is not a symptom=cure sort of healing technique. It involves a careful study of the defensive abilities of each individual patient's body. Practitioners have to have the knowledge to differentiate between disease symptoms and the defensive or recovery systems.

What Holism believes is that when someone falls sick, their whole body has undergone some kind of weakness and has lost the balance of its strength. So the solution is to simply restore the strength of the body.

All western natural health therapies rely on biological factors and the better developed psychosocial approaches are a modern addition.

Individualism

This concept is different in the sense that it places all responsibility for sickness and good health on every individual in a society. So everyone is responsible for their personal health.

Individualism results from an awareness of the importance of individuals in a community and the resulting virtues of self-reliance and personal independence. Well-rounded individuals are both self-reliant and independent.

Victim-blaming

What this means is that if someone gets sick then the victim of the sickness did something wrong. While it might sound a little weird what it honestly means is that personal health is a personal responsibility and no one can blame someone or something else for his or her illness. It focuses on the self. Improve yourself because the environment around you is too big to change for one individual. In other words, health problems should be self corrected and the obvious solution is a change in the victim's lifestyle.

Prevention

This is probably the most difficult concept for the modern day individual to grasp. Though everyone is aware of the phrase 'prevention is better than cure' there are few people who actually go the extent of preventing even the most obvious trouble (think about smoking, alcohol, high cholesterol foods, sugar, etc.). Prevention does not merely suggest that troublesome activities should be avoided. What is says is that improving health is better than fighting disease. It suggests the application of this to short term as well as long term negative effects. In the short term, a healthy body can easily ward off minor illnesses (like common cold) and injuries (razor cuts, skin peeling during sports activities for instance). In the long term prevention suggests caution in all that is done today so that it does not result in adverse outcomes in the future. In other words, it too suggests a change in lifestyle for a healthier tomorrow.

Reasonably good health can be achieved by everyone. What is even better that the means to do so do not have to acquired from anyone, the capacity to do so lies within us.

The next few pages focus exclusively on herbs and subsequently on natural herbal cures.

NATURAL HERBS

Any plant that is grown for culinary, medicinal, or in some cases even spiritual value is called an herb. It is common practice that, from an herb plant only the green and leafy parts are used. The culinary usages are obviously different from the medicinal uses, in fact, it is often the case that the properties of culinary and medicinal herbs are entirely different to be found in the same plant. For example, medicinal herbs usually tend to be shrubs or woody plants. Culinary herbs, on the other hand, are typically more leafy and soft.

Interestingly, the seeds, berries, bark, root, or other parts of a herbal plant make great spices. These plants also bear edible fruits or vegetables.

Culinary herbs are different from other vegetables in the sense that they are not the primary objects to be cooked or consumed. Instead, they are used to provide flavor when used as spices.

Botanical definitions

Botanical science defines a herb as a plant that does not produce a woody stem. It usually dies in temperate climates. Death can be complete in case of annual herbs or the herb can simply go back to its roots in case of perennial herbs.

Examples of herbs include: bulbs, peonies, hosta, grasses, and banana.

The botanical term herbaceous means a plant having the characteristic of a herb or being leaf-like in color and texture.

Herbalism

Herbalism is also known as phytotherapy. It is a very old folk medicine that is based on the use of plants and plant extracts. Human beings have been looking for healing powers in the vegetable kingdom for a long time. There are innumerable types of indigenous plants that have been used by people for centuries in the treatment of many ailments. The history of such usage is long and well documented. Evidence has been found that sixty thousand years ago the Neanderthals living in present day Iraq used plants as medicines.

Radiocarbon dating of the Lascaux caves in France has revealed that cave paintings dated between 13000-25000 BCE displays the use of plants as healing agents.

It must be appreciated that our forefathers spent several centuries slowly building upon the knowledge of their own predecessors to arrive at proper medical conclusions. It took many generations of trial and error to expand this knowledge base. The individuals who took upon themselves the task of following this line of reasoning and medical discovery are whom we today remember as "healers" or "Shaman".

An interesting aspect of plants is their seemingly infinite ability to synthesize aromatic substances like phenols and tannins. Plants also evolve alkaloids that serve as defense mechanisms against predatory microorganisms, insects, and herbivores. Plants and chemicals have a strong and historical relationship going back to several hundred millions of years. The chemical interactions in a plant's metabolism, offense, and defense procedures is very complex. Human beings have found that many herbs and species that are used in seasoning of good often yielded useful medical compounds.

In recent years plants have once again come into the foreground as the search for new drugs and dietary supplements have led researchers back into the plant kingdom.

Pharmacologists, microbiologists, botanists, and natural product chemists are literally going through the entire roster of plant species with a fine toothed comb looking for phytochemicals that could lead to the development of cures for several types of diseases. Already there are many drugs on the market that have been derived from plants.

Herbal treatment of diseases is nearly universal in all non-industrialized societies. Since they do not have the resources to set up pharmaceutical industries and are quite likely to be too impoverished to purchase modern day drugs, it should not be surprising that they rely on plants that they can grown to fight off illness.

In western society, the use of herbal medicine can be contributed to the cumulation of several traditions over a long stretch of time, finally culminating at the end of the twentieth century. Some of these influences are based on ancient Greek and Rome, the Ayurvedic principles from India, and Chinese herbal medicines.

Some very common plant based pharmaceuticals that have been used by western physicians include opium, aspirin, digitalis, and quinine.

Background

In any living organism, chemical reactions define the metabolism rate and control normal metabolic activities. Some of these chemicals are known as primary metabolites (sugar and fat) and are found in nearly all plants. Chemicals known as secondary metabolites are found in a limited number of plants. The functions of secondary metabolites can be very different. They could be used to produce alkaloids (poisons) for defense or to attract insects to enhance pollination.

Most of the therapeutic chemicals derived from plants as well plant- based modern drugs rely on the secondary metabolite chemicals in plants. A few examples are: inulin (roots of the plant dahlias), quinine (from cinchona), morphine and codeine (from poppy), and digoxin (from foxglove).

The National Center for Complementary and Alternative Medicine has started to fund clinical trials to improve the medical world's understanding of herbal medicine.

Popularity

In May 2004, the National Center for Complementary and Alternative Medicine conducted a survey. The focus of this survey was on people who had used Complementary and

Alternative Medicines (CAM), what particular types of treatments were used, and why did the people choose for the complementary medicine option.

The results of this survey indicated that, with the exclusion of prayer, herbal therapy (or the use of natural products besides vitamins and minerals) was the highest used complementary and alternative medicine. 18.9% opted for herbal therapy over all other forms of complementary and alternative medicines.

Here are a few samples of medicines used in herbal therapy.

- A variety of plants (including artichoke) help to reduce the total serum cholesterol levels.
- Plants like black cohosh (and others that contain phytoestrogens or active estrogen) have proven effective in treating symptoms of menopause
- A limited number of studies have reported that the average length of common cold can be reduced by using echinacea extracts.
- Garlic is a herb that provides multiple benefits like lowering of cholesterol levels, lowering blood pressures, and reducing platelet aggregation.
- Another highly diverse medicinal plant is black cumin (nigella sativa). Common ailments that can be cured

using black cumin include: cough, pulmonary infections, asthma, influenza, allergy, hypertension, and stomachache. The seeds of black cumin are classified as carminative, stimulant, diuretic, and galactogogue. Seed powder or oil from black cumin can be applied externally in case of skin eruptions.

Digestive tract problems including irritable bowel syndrome and nausea can be relieved by drinking peppermint tea.

- Rauvolfa serpentina is one of the oldest and most widely used herbs in India. It is applied for treating problems like insomnia, anxiety, and hypertension. This herb is also the foundation for the first plant based allopathic drug that was developed to combat high blood pressure.
- In some clinical trials it has been discovered that St. John's wort, a most dangerous chemical, can be highly effective in cases of mild to moderate depression
- Another plant root that can be used in the treatment of sleeplessness is valerian.

Dangers

All modern pharmaceutical drugs need to be prescribed due to dangers of side effects or allergic reactions, or possibly reaction with other drugs. This has resulted in the development of a myth about natural products, including herbalism, that has spread far and wide. The myth goes that natural products are safe. Or, anyone can take them without consulting an expert and they will do no harm.

In the end, whatever we extract from plants, spices of curative agents, we are dealing with chemicals. Over centuries the defense system of plants has led them to produce some very lethal chemicals. There are innocent looking plants that can give an adult nausea if a single leaf is smelled close closely. A small nibble of the same leaf by an infant can be fatal.

Fortunately, most such plants are found deep in the forests where predators other than man are a threat. Still, there are milder forms of toxins in plants much closer to us and even these can be lethal if caution is found lacking. For example, hemlock and nightshade are two plants that can prove to be fatal through carelessness.

Also to be remembered is the fact that plants or herbal remedies are as likely to cause side effects and allergic reactions as other pharmaceutical drugs. However, these problems usually result from improper dosage and impurities.

Another danger is taking herbal remedies with conventional drugs when both perform the same task. In that case the cumulative effect will surely result in an overdose.

Effectiveness

Scientific studies provide indisputable evidence that the herbals extracts from plants can not only cure but also prevent certain types of diseases. Further evidence of the benefits of herbal medicine can be found in the fact that there are many modern pharmaceutical drugs available that use plant extracts.

The need for caution comes in when reading the advertisements and other marketing materials for alternative medicines, even if they are plant based, 100% natural and completely safe. There are no products on the market that will advertise boldly that they might not be effective in some cases. That sort of statement is usually hidden in the small print.

That should not be criteria when choosing an alternative medication. There are cases where scientific studies have shown that people receive none of the medical benefits that the product claims to deliver. There are many alternative medicines on the market that have not undergone any sort of testing whatsoever.

The importance of scientific testing becomes apparent when you consider that these old-age natural therapy concepts were developed when there were no scientific controls and no test procedures. If someone wanted to try out a new herb, the easiest way for to try it on themselves first. Secondly, the human mind was not as well understood as it is today. For example, modern controls can easily make out the difference between a placebo effect, the body's ability to heal itself through its immune system, and the actual practical benefits of herbs.

Without this understanding any herb, whether beneficial or not, can be made to look like a life saver.

Scientific investigation also helps to reveal the precise nature and structure of the chemicals in an herb. Which chemicals do what. How to they react with blood and other internal organs. What chemical combines where to produce what compound – finally resulting in a cure or relief. These are important facets of scientific testing that were not available in the days when herbal traditions were being established. Most knowledge in those days was anecdotal and based on personal experience. Humanity and especially the medical workers know better today.

It is always prudent to choose a medical treatment that has been proven safe and effective. It is possible for people to get so influenced by the natural healing movement that they will abandon conventional medicine altogether. Avoid falling into this trap.

Herbal therapies have just begun to be studied scientifically and until proven safe and sound should only be used as complementary alternative medicines, not the main treatment.

The chemical composition of a lot of herbs is still not known so there is always the standing danger of violent reaction to an alkaloid. Do not underestimate this.

Standards

Different countries allot different legal status to different herbal ingredients. For example, ayurveda, the alternative medicine therapy from India believes that heavy metals are therapeutic. The United States however believes that high levels of heavy metals are actually unsafe for normal consumption. So ayurvedic medicines are not granted the same status as regular drugs and they are certainly not FDA approved.

Like other non-FDA-approved health products, ayurvedic drugs are sold in the United States as dietary supplements and not medicines. This is merely an evasion because as per American laws, supplements do not need to be tested for safety or effectiveness. In some cases even quality control of the active ingredients can be inadequate.

Usage

If you intend to use herbal remedies then it is always advisable to first have a detailed and frank discussion with your doctor. Keep in mind that herbal remedies can cause adverse reactions just like conventional drugs. This risk is augmented when herbal remedies are taken in combination with prescription or over the counter drugs. For example, if you are taking medication for hypertension (these medicines lower blood pressure) and at the same time you take a herbal supplement with the same affect, there is a very high risk possibility of blood pressure dropping dangerously.

There are also many supplements available that might contain herbs, which are to be strictly avoided during pregnancy.

HERBOLOGY

Herbology is the name given to the Chinese method of combining medicinal herbs. In this technique, which is one of the most widely used in Traditional Chinese Medicine (TCM), every herbal medicine is actually a cocktail of several herbs that are customized to individual patients. The doctor will assess the yin/yang condition of a patient in addition to studying the symptoms of the ailment.

The preparation of the medicine begins with the use of or two main herbs that target the ailment. The other herbs are added in order to adjust the yin/yang condition. Other ingredients can be added to cancel out toxicity or side effects resulting from the main herbs.

This sort of herbal mixing to arrive at a formula that is suitable to individual needs is not easy. A lot of experience and tutelage is required before a practicing of traditional Chinese medicine can perform the mixing independently.

An important difference between traditional Chinese medicine and modern drugs is that the balance and chemical interaction of the ingredients a formula is considered more important than the individual ingredients.

Another quirk in Chinese herbology is that while it may be called herbology it will use all parts of a plant including: leaf, stem, flower, root. In fact, some remedies will also use ingredients derived from animals and minerals. This has caused quite a bit of controversy because sometimes traditional Chinese medicine can call for ingredient from animals that are declared as endangered species (seahorses, rhinoceros, tigers, etc.).

Shennong is usually considered to be the first Chinese herbalist. It is said that Shennong tasted hundreds of herbs and experimented with them before passing on his knowledge of medicinal and poisonous plants to the farmers of China. He also wrote the first Chinese manual on pharmacology: the Shennong Bencao Jing. This manual lists approximately 365 medicines out of which 252 are herbal. The manual is dated around the 1st century Han dynasty.

One of the most important of such documents that were written by several master practitioners of Chinese herbology is the Bencao Gangmu. It was put together by Li Shizhen during the Ming dynasty. The contents of Bencao Gangmu are so potent that even today they are used for consultation and reference.

Classification of Chinese herbs is in itself a very intricate process. Very broadly speaking, Chinese herbs are classified using methods such as those described below.

The Four Natures

The four natures are basically the yin and yang states and how effective a herbal medication is in bringing them into balance. Yin and yang degrees can range from cold (extreme yin), cool, neutral (warm), or hot (extreme yang). Before selecting herbs the doctor will make a careful study of the yin/yang balance in a patient. So if the patient has "internal cold" then an herb that has a "hot" yang value will be used and so on.

The Five Tastes

Some herbs are identified by their taste. While the taste in itself has no medicinal value in the absence of a better yardstick Chinese medicine associates the taste associated with an herb to the final effect. These five tastes are pungent, sweet, sour, bitter, and salty.

Each taste has its own function. Pungent herbs are used to increase sweating, vitalizing blood and Qi. Sweet herbs are used to tone and harmonize body systems. Other sweet herbs help in curing excessive dampness by way of diuresis. Sour taste is meant to be astringent. Bitter tasting herbs help the body get rid of excess heat, empty the bowels, and reduce dampness by causing dryness. Salty herbs can help to soften up hard masses.

The Meridians

Meridians do not have anything to do with the Earth's meridians or magnetism. What they refer to is the precise organ that the chemicals in a herb target. So menthol which is pungent and cool is associated with lungs and liver. This means that since lungs are the organs that protect the body from cold and influenza the use of menthol can help to get rid of coldness in the lungs and also resist heat toxins.

ALTERNATIVE NATURAL HERBAL CURES

Herbs today are being increasing used to treat all kinds of disorders. From mild cases like common cold to serious diseases like cancer, there is an ever growing need for genuine and well tested information regarding herbal cures.

The information, in a rudimentary way, has already been gathered for us a long time ago. While most of this knowledge precedes modern scientific thinking, the integration of the two needs careful execution.

Long past civilizations in places like the Indus valley (in the Indian subcontinent) have left us with many concepts like holistic approach, righteous living, yoga, meditation, etc. As far as medicine goes, from the same location appeared Ayurveda that defined proper diagnosis and herbal cures for several diseases.

Thanks to the Internet and the world wide web there is practically no limit to the number of websites that are busy claiming that they have managed to master age old secrets or discovered some long lost magic cure to end all human suffering. There are also some saner websites that are more lucid and honest about their claims. However, there are no proper medical outlets for these cures. They are all businesses with the only objective of making profits. This makes it very difficult for the average person to know whom they can trust when considering herbal remedies.

Sadly, due to the misguided media propagation of herbal medicines there is a gold rush of sorts that involves people who wish to capitalize on the growing popularity of herbal medicines and supplements with no regard as to its scientific or personal implications.

This immoral approach has in turn brought a lot of negative publicity for herbal treatment as the voice of genuine scientists is drowned in the fraudulent claims of businesses. Hydrotherapy was a good idea but how can anyone take it seriously when it is so closely associated with sale of "colored water"?

If you have been brought to cultivate a negative image of herbal medicine then try to remember a simple thing. Medical science is several thousand years old and while there have been several blunders in that time, herbal medication has been helping people through countless generations. There are genuine herbal cures out there. Do not give in to the advertised products but speak to your doctor.

HERBAL MEDICINE CURES

One of the oldest forms of health care that has been with humanity is herbal medicine. All over the world, across several cultures, history is rife with evidence that our predecessors used herbs for medicinal purposes. This should not come as a surprise because herbs, unlike modern medicine, are usually safe and do not involve as many side effects.

The late twentieth century saw a reemergence of herbal remedies with the popular of herb-based medications increasing dramatically. More and more hospitals are now offering herbal remedies as complementary alternative treatments with conventional medicines. With this increase in public acceptance of herbal remedies, it has become imperative to conduct studies that can help medical science to understand how herbal medicine works by interacting chemically with our internal bodily functions.

Though it is normally true that herbs and medications derived from them produce fewer side effects than many allopathic medicines taken for similar symptoms, it is important to remember that even plants contain certain chemicals that can produce toxicity after long-term use. Also, while plant based medicines are usually safe even they can be abused. Unlike allopathic medicines that have trouble staying in the body for extended periods, herbal chemicals can create residues in the body and over a long time this slow poisoning can lead to sickness that cannot be diagnosed or even death.

Just like other medications and food supplements there is always the condition and body type of the individual to be considered before prescribing anything. Many health conditions and complications make it necessary for people with those problems to avoid certain types of herbal medicine.

Ask any doctor, they will tell you that it is a very bad and risky idea to mix medications. In certain cases, this applies to herbal medicines as well. They should never be mixed with other herbs (or extracts) and medications. When hospitals offer herbal therapies as complimentary alternative treatments they make certain that the reaction of the herbs will not conflict with the main course of medication administered. This is not something you should mix and match at home. Consult your doctor before making a medicinal cocktail. Obviously, should you notice any symptoms that ring your internal warning bell, please rush to your doctor immediately.

One of the things that people often do wrong is attempt to self- diagnose minor ailments. This is a classic medical trap that most medical students learn very early. Symptoms are so easy to misread that it is common for people to assume that the minor problem they have is actually some serious, life threatening issue. Conversely, bad reading of serious symptoms as being related to some minor problem instead of the real thing is equally dangerous. Do not attempt to self-diagnose if you are not from a medical background and even then, be very careful.

Trying a treatment without understanding the problem will most likely create a whole slew of problems that you never had before.

Do not assume that just because you are taking herbs then it does not matter because they will not harm you anyway. Precautions are necessary even with relatively harmless medications.

Since herbal medicines have not been properly scrutinized, the values attributed to them are based on broad generalized descriptions that originated thousands of years ago. Ancient texts explain a lot of things but do not actually tell us how herbal medicine works. We just know through experience and observation that they do. In light of this, it becomes difficult to determine beforehand certain medicinal puzzles like:

- What can be the possible side effects
- What internal complications/medication conflicts can create problems
- What is the maximum and minimum range for a safe dose for a specific patient
- How many different herbs should be there in each dose
- How does a patient or healer know that an overdose has happened

It is impossible to know how safe a particular herbal mixture is unless you know precisely the exact contents of the mixture along with a breakdown in terms of the number of herbs and the proportional content of each herb. Simply taking too much of it in the hopes that things will work out for the best is a dangerous choice to follow because of certain toxic side effects of the chemicals in herbal medicines.

Certain cases were reported in the past where a lack of understanding, like the points listed above, or worse, an overwhelming underestimation of the potency of herbal medicines had caused the medical conditions of people to worsen by several degrees. Some of these people underwent hospitalized, not for their original ailment but just to treat the side effects of improperly administered herbal medicine. Thanks to the modern media hype surrounding natural products as opposed to industrially manufactured ones, there has developed a tendency for developed nations to think that "natural" and "safe" are synonymous. They are nothing of the sort and it would be prudent to avoid that particular confusion.

All this should not discourage you or cause you to look at herbal medicine as something practiced by quacks and fraught with danger. As mentioned earlier, this healing technique has been around for a long, long time and has mostly benefited humanity. When there has been a problem, it has been due to incompetent judgment on part of the healer or an overdose by the patient. With a little care and discretion, anyone can take herbal supplements or medicines.

CHINESE HERBAL MEDICINE

One of the oldest cultures that carried out a thorough study of herbs and other plant life related to human health was ancient China.

Chinese Herbal Medicine, also referred to as CHM, went through many evolutions, as the knowledge grew more and more refined. Remember that the nature of illnesses that afflict humanity change over time. Over the thousands of years that CHM was, so to speak, in development, the nature of these afflictions changed and CHM had to change its mode of thinking and conduct more research to combat new invasions of the human body. Chinese hospitals use all the advantages offered by modern medicinal research and techniques while at the same time they rely on their ages old CHM to treat many diseases and disorders.

Chinese Herbal Medicine claims that it can cure any kind of disease. This claim is good when you consider that CHM

44

takes the preventative approach rather than the curative one. CHM first tries to make sure that no disease can affect the body and in case it does, early detection makes preventative cures possible. However, even Chinese Herbal Medicine can do little against a problem like third- stage cancer.

After pharmaceutical drugs, a majority of the world population uses Chinese Herbal Medicine as a first alternative. CHM also produces fewer side effects when compared to mainstream pharmaceutical drugs.

The duration of treatment using CHM depends on the type of disease and its severity. Therefore, there is no predefined period of treatment. It is customized to be shorter or longer as needed.

Some common ailments that can be treated with the help of CHM are allergies, digestion problems, problems resulting from respiratory tract complications, immune system disorders, many types of pains (internal and external), psychological disorders and fallout problems, most diseases that afflict children and infants, an assortment of gynecological complications.

There is no particular age limit applicable to the use of Chinese Herbal Medicine. Nor is there any restriction based on personal constitutions. However, like any form of treatment, it is best to know of existing symptoms and previous medical history (especially relating to medicinal conflicts and reactions, or allergies) that need due consideration before even a dose of CHM is prescribed. Other than that, there is no problem in prescribing Chinese Herbal Medicine to pregnant women or women who are breast-feeding. Of course, a lot depends on what is being prescribed.

Chinese Herbal Medicines are available in different forms and there is the choice between traditional CHM and the modernized versions. Some people find it difficult to adjust to the peculiar taste of CHM but just keep at it and it will soon become acceptable.

There is no standard pricing scheme for CHM and so you might have to fish a bit to find the right price. Also, note that recently insurance companies have started covering herbal treatment. So if you are into herbal medicines have yet to take out an insurance policy you might want to investigate this possibility with your insurance provider.

One way Chinese Herbal Medicine does its magic is by removing excess toxins from the body. This is done in many ways. One method is the colonic dialysis therapy. This therapy is especially effective with people who are trying to overcome addictions. While the human body gathers toxins from all sorts of sources on a daily basis, addictions result in rapid toxin build up in a very short time. What is worse, depending on the type of addiction, natural toxin excretion from the body is inhibited. Colonic dialysis therapy overcomes these inhibitions and provides a quick exit route for the accumulated toxins. For people who are blessed enough to escape addictions the natural toxin release mechanism is given a boost by colonic dialysis therapy.

Currently the PLA Institute of Drug Dependence Treatment and Rehabilitation is busy doing earnest research to study how colonic dialysis therapy can help people who have been long-term addicts of heroin. The primary focus of this research is to determine whether colonic dialysis therapy helps these people to abstain from heroin and whether it can reduce craving and the resulting withdrawal symptoms.

The doctors of the Royal Free Hospital, London, carried out another scientific study of Chinese Herbal Medicine. In this study, Chinese remedies were evaluated for the help they might offer to dermatitis patients. About ten different types of herbs were mixed together to create the "cure" that was being tested. This mixture was then given to forty adult patients who had a long medical history of coping with atopic dermatitis (commonly known as eczema). The evaluation period lasted for five months. During an eight-week period in this study, patients

47

were randomly given either the mixture that was being tested or a placebo that tasted and looked just the same. This is normally done so that patient responses can be monitored under blind circumstances. Out of the forty patients, thirty-one stayed through the entire course of the study and they all displayed continuous and rapid improvement in erythema (redness of skin caused by eczema). Obviously, the study concluded that Chinese Herbal Medicine was an effective remedy for adult atopic dermatitis.

DIFFERENT TYPES
OF HERBAL MEDICINE

There are many positive aspects that herbal medicine has going for it. Unfortunately, the lack of adequate scientific understanding means that there is no way a doctor can completely take responsibility for what is being prescribed and hence the safety factor involved in taking herbal medicines is suspect.

The drugs that we normally take have to undergo thorough testing and need FDA approval. This entire process ensures that every single chemical in the medicine and its interaction with the human body (and resulting side effects) are well understood, documented, and scientifically demonstrable.

While herbal medicines enjoy the reputation of being less complicated it should be remembered that they are manufactured by Mother Nature and she does not need FDA approval or scientific testing.

Fortunately, thousands of years of development have put herbal medicines into a certain safety zone that has helped many a human being with being cured.

So herbal medicines might be risky but there is no need to worry if you take the simple precaution of consulting your doctor before consuming any herbal concoction Doctors are sort of walking pharmacopoeias and they know more about all those chemicals and stuff. They can advise you properly.

Another thing to know with herbal medicine is that different cultures have resulted in different types of herbal therapies.

Finally, thanks to the Internet and online marketing there is no shortage of frauds selling roots and leaves grown in their backyards. Make certain that when you get herbal medicine it comes from genuine herbs. The wrong herbs might possibly contain toxic chemicals that make a trip to the hospital inevitable.

Some common forms of herbal medicines are as follows:

- Essence. You have probably come across the line "essence of ..." followed by some plant or flower when reading an ad for a cosmetic product. While Essences tend to get associated with cosmetic products due to massive advertising of those products, certain essential oils are always available for therapeutic purposes. The popularity of essential herbal oils processed through cold pressing or steam distillation is because many people prefer to get a massage than eating a pill. The most common benefit of essential oils is the help they provide in relaxing. They do not really cure any problems. Their major effect is to provide relief.

- Body massages can release toxins in the muscles, aiding relaxation.

- Head massages can likewise reduce heaviness or, in some cases, cure headaches. Similarly, chest massages using essence of certain herbs can help with congestion resulting from common cold.

- Pills or capsules. There was a time when this alternative was not available. It was a dark time for people who could not stand the taste of raw herbal medicines. The pills and capsules were a godsend for people who wanted to try herbal remedies but were unable to swallow. In order to convert a herb to pill form it first needs to be dried and crushed into powder. What is of interest is that there are hardly any herbal medicines available in pill or capsule form that target specific ailments. They act more like secondary medications to provide moral support to whatever primary medication is being taken. Professionals in herbal medicine believe that the drying and crushing of the herbs robs them of their potency. Others suggest that herbal medicine should be taken in its raw form for complete effectiveness. Anyway, if you are looking for specific herbal medicines instead of general health enhancers and supplements then this option is not for you.

- Infusions. The most popular form of herbal infusion is the drinking of various kinds of tea. Infusion involves the use of the delicate parts (leaves, seeds, and fruits) of a herbal plant and are quick to administer. Some ingredients of infusion tea could be stinging nettle, oat straw, red clover, raspberry leaf, and comfrey leaf. Infusions can be just the tea you drink normally (but using herbs instead of tealeaves) or what is, known as Medicinal Strength Tea. Most herbal teas fall into this category though the preparation is slightly different. There are several recipes available on the Internet for making Medicinal Strength Tea.

- Poultice. For injuries, inflammations, cramps, or other spasmodic problems it can become necessary to apply the herbal mixture as a poultice. The required herbs are first macerated or chopped into small pieces. These are then applied directly to the affected area and covered with a hot and moist bandage. In some cases, the herbal mixture can be applied as a layer to the moist bandage before wrapping it around the affected area.

- Raw. As the name suggests, in this case the herbal medicine is taken in its most natural form without any additives or changes to make it palatable. Most people will run a mile in tight shoes to avoid this form of medication. It is the equivalent of taking a regular capsule, pulling it open, taking that powder, putting it on the tongue and trying to suck on it as if it were chocolate. Not done, well at least not if the taste buds are functioning normally. No wonder this method in unpopular. The good news is that most of the herbs that need to be taken raw can alternatively be soaked (or passed through) water to make medicinal strength teas, and those are, much easier on sensitive palates. It is also believed that teas increase the effectiveness of raw herbs,

- Tinctures. There are very few kids who get exposed to this form of medicine these days but about twenty odd years ago no kid that got into a scrap in the field escaped the terror of tincture. These are basically herbal medicines in a liquid form. They can be for external as well as internal use. Modern incarnations are a lot milder that their older forms.

- Decoctions. A decoction is a liquid preparation made by boiling a medicinal plant with water usually in the proportion of 5 parts of the drug to 100 parts of water. Typically, certain specific parts of a plant like berries, roots, and herb-bark are used in this process. Depending on the consistency of the plant part being used, it can take up to two hours to prepare a decoction. This process extracts the flavor and increases the concentration of the herb through the process of boiling.

That more or less covers the different types of herbal medicines available. Depending on your requirement and personal taste you might need to take them in one of the above forms.

HERBAL DIET SUPPLEMENTS

Herbal supplements are a type of dietary supplement that contain herbs. An herb (also known as a botanical) is a plant or plant part used for its scent, flavor, and therapeutic properties.

Diet supplements derived from herbs usually contain more than one type of herb. The purpose of an herbal diet supplement is to increase the benefits that you get from your normal diet and to ward off the negative effects. Herbal diet supplements are rich in vitamins, minerals, amino acids, etc. Obviously, dietary supplements are not meant to be used as treatments or cures of any disease or medical condition. They are more effective as preventative agents that help strengthen the body and the immune system to naturally ward off any infections or internal malfunctions. For people who do not manage a balanced diet herbal diet supplements also supply necessary nutrients missing from regular diet.

Many herbal dietary supplements can provide substantial aid for different types of medical conditions.

Some herbal diet supplements are:

• **Ephedra**. This supplement increases the body resistance towards common cold, helps in the treatment of asthma and upper respiratory problems. For people who work out regularly, ephedra is an important ingredient in most fat loss supplements.

• **Magnesium**. Minerals and salts are the biggest deficiencies in an unbalanced diet. Magnesium is essential in preventing kidney, thyroid, and heart disease. There are many herbal diet supplements rich in magnesium.

• **St. John's wort.** Also known as hypericum, Klamath weed, and goat weed, this supplement has been used for centuries in the treatment of mental disorders, nerve pain. In older times it was also used as a sedative and malaria cure. Nowadays, the common uses are treatment of depression, anxiety, and sleep disorders. It is typically consumed as a tea or in pill form.

• **Vitamin E.** Uncontrolled oxidation in our body can result in long-term damage. That is why our bodies generate anti-oxidants. However, if the production of anti-oxidants falls below safe levels then external supplements are required.

- **One very potent anti-oxidant is vitamin E**. Herbal diet supplements rich in vitamin E make good anti-oxidants.

- **Copper**. While metals and minerals are essential to the normal functioning of our body, sometimes they can fail to get absorbed properly. Zinc is essential for our body and there is nothing better than a copper rich herbal diet supplement. These supplements increase the absorption of zinc. The result is better protection against heart disease, and healthier skin and hair color.

- **Folate**. From a certain viewpoint, folates are required more than anything else because they can affect us down to our DNA. Folates are required for the production and maintenance of new cells (especially during pregnancy and infancy). DNA replication cannot take place without folates. Folates also prevent cancer causing DNA changes. Folate deficiency affects the bone marrow where most new cells are produced. Folates are needed to make new red blood cells and prevent anemia. As you can see, any deficiency in folates can be devastating in the end. One of the earliest indications of folate deficiency is anemia. Herbal diet supplements that have folates as major ingredients are always good for you, even if you do not have any problem currently.

- **Iron**. In the human body, the metal iron is more pervasive than any other. It plays an important part in several vital functions. Iron carries oxygen to the lungs and muscles in the form of hemoglobin. It acts as a means of transport for electrons between cells. It is a catalyst for enzyme reactions in tissues. Iron deficiency most commonly occurs in children and pre-menopausal women. It can easily prove to be fatal if left unchecked. Herbal diet supplements rich in iron can help to prevent such a situation.

- **Vitamin B6 and B12.** Vitamin B6 (pyridoxine) deficiency can lead to anemia, depression, dermatitis, and high blood pressure. Vitamin B12 (cyanocobalamin) deficiency can lead to anemia, memory loss, and cognitive decline. It is most likely to occur among elderly people. In extreme cases it can even cause paralysis can result. It is widely used in the treatment of alcoholism, depression, diabetes, hair loss, and stress. Vegans are especially at risk of B12 deficiency because vitamin B12 naturally occurs only in meats. So if you are a vegan than an herbal dietary supplement with vitamins B6 and B12 is an absolute must for you.

- **Tea**. Most herbal teas (and especially Medicinal Strength Teas) involve the use of herbs that have anti-oxidant properties useful in prevention of cancer, heart disease, high blood pressure. Since these teas usually do not involve caffeine and other associated chemicals they are better from a health perspective than regular tea or coffee.

- **Vitamin D**. The human body (especially skin) develops its own vitamin D. It is necessary to maintain normal levels of calcium and phosphorous. A direct result of vitamin D deficiency is a weaker skeleton, a condition known as osteoporosis where the bones become porous and hence break easily. Vitamin D herbal supplements can help prevent osteoporosis.

- **Selenium**. This is a chemical so volatile that it does not occur in its free state in nature. Toxic in large amounts, trace amounts of it form the center of some enzymes that are vital to the normal working of all cells in nearly all living organisms. In the human body it behaves as an anti-oxidant and is also important for the normal working of the thyroid gland. Cereals, meat, fish, and eggs are good sources of selenium. Since the majority of sources are animal based, vegans and vegetarians should seriously herbal dietary supplements containing selenium.

- **Vitamin A**. This vitamin is responsible for maintaining good eye sight and promoting bone growth. It is also an anti-oxidant. Most skin and eye problems are related to vitamin A deficiency so if you have any such conditions, consider a herbal diet supplement rich in vitamin A.

ADVANTAGES
OF HERBAL DIET SUPPLEMENTS

Here is a crash course in the advantages of herbal supplements and medicines:

- **They are cheap**. Did you look at your medical bills for the past year? Now add up all that you paid the pharmacist for prescription and over-the-counter medications. Is the number looking scary yet? So if you have been using conventional medicine for small problems like common cold and stomachaches then perhaps it is time you considered herbal medicine. It might give you a healthier wallet or purse besides a healthy body.

- **You can do it**. Did you know that herbal medicine and supplements can be assembled in your own kitchen? There are thousands of herbal recipes available on the Internet. Just follow them like a recipe to bake a cake and there you are. Your medicine made by your own hand. If you have a garden you could even grown your own herbs.

- **They are natural.** Man has learned to do many things but nature continues to know more. So matter how much noise the pharmaceutical companies make you should at least give some time to listen to nature and her own remedies.

Now for the long version.

Herbal medicines, therapies, and supplements are nothing new. People have used them for centuries but it is only recently that western culture has rediscovered the wonders of herbs. In part, this was because the development of allopathic medicinal techniques in the west combined with the lack of scientific support for non- conventional medicines to give an unsavory (and quite wrong) reputation to herbal medicines and supplements. Recent discoveries have forced the medical community to reconsider the benefits of herbs. This has mostly come about with increasing exposure of western community to the healing techniques practiced in other cultures and countries that proved to be more effective than, or at the least complimentary to, allopathic treatment.

People were falling sick a long time ago and even they needed something to help ease the pain and maybe do away with the cause altogether. In the absence of modern medical techniques, they turned to the only things they had around them: plants and herbs. Soon they were busy treating everything from stomachaches to depression and insomnia.

Modern medical science is discovering that these simply remedies from the distant past are not without merit and when combined with a healthy lifestyle and present day rules of personal hygiene, they can really be a potent force in preventing illness and promoting general good health and well-being. Since they do not involve some of the more serious side effects of conventional medicine these herbal supplements can be taken for a variety of preventative reasons. For example, some herbal supplements help lower cholesterol, enhance memory performance, improve the quality of mental concentration, strengthen the cardiovascular system, and increase energy and stamina.

There was a time when food had to travel a very short distance. Grains arrived quickly from the farmer, milk and bacon came fresh from the milkman, most people had gardens to grow their own plants. Those were the days without preservatives and fertilizers and, hard as it may be, people were a lot healthier back then. The reason is that massive production and manufacturing pressures inevitably result in poor handling and use of artificial preservatives. Due to this, a lot of the food that we eat today is lacking in important vitamins, minerals, and other essential nutrients before it even appears on the shelves. No matter how healthy the label claims the food inside to be, fresh is fresh, and preservatives mean loss of food quality for the sake of profits. A normal diet comprised of the same elements will leave you deficient in several important nutrients if it is not fresh.

This is one reason why herbal dietary supplements have suddenly become important today and are being studied so closely by the medical community. They are safe, they are as close to natural and fresh as they get, and they are the most effective means available to the common people to ensure that their body has all the required types of fuel to keep it going at maximum efficiency day after day even in the face of improper diets.

A note of caution is in order here to warn you that since herbal supplements are not subject to government regulations or general scrutiny it is quite natural that there are some very ill-minded people out there who are putting up substandard products to cash in on the herbal medicine and supplement craze. It is vital to avoid these products, as the total harm they will end up doing is unjustifiable against the limited good they might do. When you go shopping for herbal products, do a thorough research of the company manufacturing them. You are shopping for your health so make certain that it is safe from malicious products and greedy corporations. Look out for Certificate of Analysis (COA) for each ingredient in the supplement. Also make certain that the manufacturing company follows the GMP manufacturing processes strictly. In the absence of regulations similar to those that apply to pharmaceutical companies, GMP is the best you can hope for from a company manufacturing herbal products.

Nowadays you do not need to go down to the local health store to purchase nutritional health supplements.

Just connect to the Internet and there are countless websites from where you cannot only purchase products online but you can also perform extensive research. Researching products is a good idea.

Do a web-search for reviews of people or visit forums where such products are discussed.

People will be more than willing to exchange posts on a personal basis on those boards.

While herbal supplements are sold as individual products it is a good idea to look for comprehensive formulae that involve different herbal extracts along with a healthy dose of vitamins, minerals, amino acids, and cofactors. Try to treat your herbal supplement as a balanced that should have a bit of everything while staying on the safe side.

Most importantly, before you make a purchase, take a print out of the details of the product that interests you and discuss it thoroughly with your doctor. Some herbal supplements might be more useful for you and conversely you might be about to spend money on supplements you do not need in the least. Your doctor can help with the practical details.

Herbal supplements are growing popular day by day. People all over the world are always looking for ways to improve their health and more and more of them are turning to natural remedies rather than the mainstream drugs that have been around for most of recent history.

Due to this increasing trend, scientists have finally decided to conduct studies to determine the therapeutic benefits and applications of the different herbs and their extracts that are used in herbal therapies and supplements. A majority of results from these experiments strongly indicate that taking herbal supplements along with maintaining a healthy lifestyle and good diet can be greatly beneficial to general health.

This is the reason why many people prefer natural health supplements. The trouble comes from the fact that like other nutritional supplements, herbal supplements are not regulated in the United States. Therefore, the manufacturers do not have to make any assurance of the safety and effectiveness of their products. They are not even required to reveal the ingredients in a health product.

One outcome of this is that a product can claim to contain a herb but a manufacturer can easily put in a chemical equivalent. This might sound criminal but unfortunately in modern corporate culture of "profits first", it is quite a normal occurrence.

The use of dietary supplements saw a dramatic increase in the 1990s but since then the use of such supplements has gone into a decline. The slight correction in this downward trend is attributed to the introduction of herbal supplements into mainstream multivitamin products.

Within the last decade the use of alternative medicines, and herbal products in particular, has increased considerably.

In the year 2001, Americans spent almost $4.2 billion on herbal and botanical remedies. This coincided with extensive media coverage of the benefits that people were enjoying from herbal remedies.

The percentage of people who were using dietary supplements increased from 14.2% (1998) to 18.8% (2002), with the low spot of 12.3% in 2000 and the highest peak at 19.8% in 2001.

The number of people ages 45-64 who were taking supplements increased by 50% between 1998-99 and 2001-02.

Broadly speaking it was discovered that the majority of people taking dietary supplements were older and mostly female (59.9% as compared to 55.5% of males).

There are many reasons for this increase, not the least being that herbal supplements do in fact being many benefits with them.

People can take herbs and supplements for any number of reasons. There are herbs like Echinacea that are extremely helpful in case of common cold or flu. If you feel constantly lethargic even when there is no weakness in the body then perhaps Ginseng tea can help to give you a boost of energy instead of a cappuccino. Ginseng can also increase sexual stamina, reduce stress levels, and fight against aging effects like memory loss.

Herbal medicine is varied and within its diversity it covers a broad range of conditions where it can be effectively applied for treatment. Furthermore, these treatments are conducted on several different levels that can range from generic every day problems that need nothing more than symptomatic relief to completely customized prescriptions that are prepared for individual conditions in patients that have undergone extensive analysis and examination at the hands of an experienced medical herbalist.

Some herbals remedies do not require consulting a qualified medical herbalist. Minor problems like mild infections, cold, cough, catarrh, stomach cramps or gas, indigestion, constipation, etc. can be cured with self-help using over the counter herbal remedies.

Self-medication using herbal remedies has never been easier thanks to the limitless information that is available today, mostly though the Internet. All it needs is a little investment of time in order to peruse these websites and anyone can make an informed decision without having to visit a medical herbalist.

In the 10th century, Arabs invented a process of distillation for the extraction of essential oils from plants. These oils were inhaled as aromas, drunk as potions, and worn aromatic amulets. This is one of the first uses of aromas as personal scent preference. This is allegedly the root behind the use of perfumes and modern day deodorants. Nowadays, this extraction process is mainly used to get the oil from plants and flowers for use in aromatherapy. This form of therapy that involves nothing more than deep inhalation of different types of herbal oils is being used to treat a wide spectrum of maladies, both physical and emotional. Headaches, herpes, dry skin, acne, arthritis, and asthma are just a few examples of the problems that people have cured using aromatherapy.

Recently, France and England started the process of reintroducing the various ancient healing techniques to the western world. This began in 1990 and aromatherapy gained a wider acceptance in the traditional community since that time.

France remains the world leader in rediscovering modern uses for ancient healing techniques. Several prominent French doctors prescribe aromatic remedies as a matter of routine for most of their patients. A visit to most French pharmacies will reveal that all of them are well stocked in a wide array of essential oils. Insurance companies in France are more than willing to pay for treatments involving aromatherapy and other traditional methods.

ARE THEIR ANY SIDE EFFECTS
TO NATURAL CURES?

A scientific study has found that, though for the most part herbal supplements seem harmless, some of the more popular products pose a very special risk. This particular supplement interacts with and reduces the effectiveness of the drug saquinavir. The only thing to do for the moment is to avoid taking herbal supplements if you are being treated with saquinavir.

Herbal supplements are meant to boost our immune system, provide more ready energy, and improve general health. Though scientists say that research that is more extensive is required to determine which herbal supplements can have an adverse effect on our body, or, can interact with other medications and reduce their effectiveness, they remain united in their stand that several of the so-called harmless supplements can prove very harmful.

Some of the more popular herbal supplements are chondroitin, ephedra, Echinacea, and glucosamine.

Chondroitin is typically used in the treatment of osteoarthritis. One side effect of chondroitin can be bleeding complications. This is more like when used in combination with a regular prescription drug that causes blood thinning.

Ephedra used to be a big favorite among people looking for a fat loss supplement. Ephedra promotes weight loss, provides energy boosts, and can also be used to treat respiratory tract problems like asthma and bronchitis. Recently, the FDA banned Ephedra because of dangerous side effects like high blood pressure, increased heart rate, false increase in metabolism, all which could lead to a cardiac arrest, heart arrhythmia, stroke, and might even be fatal in some cases.

Echinacea helps in the prevention and treatment of viral, bacterial, and fungal infections. It also helps in curing chronic wounds, ulcers, and arthritis. On the other hand it can cause immunosuppression that will cause the body to lose its self-healing capacity so wounds will not heal on their own. Immunosuppression also reduces the effectiveness of the immune system making infection easier.

Glucosamine is very often administered along with chondroitin. It contains chemicals that mimic the function of insulin and can cause the body to misbehave when this artificial insulin enters the blood stream. It can be especially bad for diabetics.

Other herbals supplements suspected of adverse side effects include gingko biloba, goldenseal, milk thistle, ginseng, kava, and garlic. It is highly advisable to seek the consultation of your doctor before taking any supplements, herbal or otherwise. More than informing you about potential health risks the doctor can give valuable advice about food, nutrition, and supplements.

AYURVEDA

Ayurvedic cures are based on ancient formulae that have been written down in the ancient Ayurvedic traditions. The success of an Ayurvedic cure depends on the quality of its ingredients.

Looking to plants for healing powers is an old idea and was embraced by the early physicians in ancient India. Ayurveda is an alternative herbal medicine therapy from India that believes heavy metals are therapeutic. The FDA considers heavy metals very dangerous for consumption and that is why Ayurvedic medicines are sold as supplements rather than medicines in America. Ayurveda is one of the oldest of traditional medicine that first established the routine of proper diagnosis and herbal cures for several diseases.

Natural Herbal Nutrition Supplements

People who opt for natural supplements or a whole food diet usually also wish to include whole food vitamins. Natural herb based supplements are usually lacking in certain vitamins that are only found in the animal kingdom so including a vitamin supplement is a wise decision. There are many companies making these vitamin supplements. One reason to prefer whole good vitamins is that they are not manufactured in a factory; they are as close to the natural form as it is possible for a packed product to be.

When you go shopping for whole food vitamins, pay close attention and make sure you do not purchase products that have preservatives or additives. Some people might also prefer their supplements in liquid form. In case a healthcare professional recommends you take supplements then it is your duty to make certain that the product you purchase is 100% natural and contains no synthetic chemicals. It is common for whole food products to contain a combination of vitamins, minerals, and other essential nutrients. You are not likely to find a whole food product that contains just one specific vitamin or mineral.

Eating whole foods and taking natural whole food vitamins is a good idea because they help to maintain healthy cells. Due to environmental pollution there are too many free radicals floating about that can easily cause cellular damage. Whole foods in all shapes can help repair that damage. Another healthy option is to include as many raw diets as you possibly can. Nowadays, thanks to pesticides, preservatives, chemical treatments, and other processes that are inflicted on foodstuff to make them healthier typically kill off a considerable proportion of important vitamins and nutrients. When you finally get these to your kitchen, the raw food is already deficient in nourishment. Cooking only makes matters worse by washing away even more vitamins and minerals. Eating a raw diet ensures that you get the maximum out of your food. A raw diet will make you feel healthier.

The New Trend?

Despite the increase in popularity that alternative medicine and herbal therapy are enjoying since the late 20th century there are opponents to the belief that these alternatives are better than conventional medicines. The growing number of adherents to the alternative therapies and herbal remedies nicely balances this out. These people have made the choice to lead a completely drug free life. According to them, even the legally manufactured and sold products by pharmaceutical companies are unhealthy because of their synthetic chemical base.

This trend is getting more widespread because nowadays there are more and more celebrities and rich public figures who are adopting the drug free lifestyle. These prominent examples prefer the use of alternative remedies for even simple problems like headaches, pains, and cramps. They steadfastly refuse the use of conventional medications and would not casually take an Advil or Aspirin because of their firm belief in the inherent health benefits that come from a drug free lifestyle.

Since herbal cures and remedies have been around for several millennia, it should not be surprising that the list of ailments they can cure and the number of cures they offer is exhaustive. There are wide arrays of symptoms, diseases, mental problems, and some physical deformities (acne), or embarrassing conditions like bad breath that can be effectively cured or greatly improved through the use of herbal remedies.

And, after all, why not? Don't you ever wonder where prescription drugs and medications come from? Everything has to have its roots in nature. There are no alien supplied medications. Every drug available on the market today once used natural substances. This changed when chemical synthesis in a factory led to rapid drug production. This was good because more people could be treated quickly and it made some pharmaceutical companies very rich. It turned out to be bad because those same pharmaceutical companies now refuse to acknowledge their roots in nature or to try and give some respectability to their parent science. Also, note that the same product when it is in a natural state requires less processing by the body as compared to its manufactured equivalent. Natural products also tend to leave behind fewer toxins in the body and are therefore better than artificial products.

A little bit of skepticism is only natural when it comes to abandoning a lifetime of faith and dependence in pharmaceutical drugs. What should be considered is the ever-increasing number of people who are adopting the herbal and natural way of life and actually benefiting from its outcome. The fact that there are some bad companies out there putting out unreliable natural and herbal products only increases the skepticism.

The marketplace is so bad today that on an average for every good product that are at leas two or three competing and thoroughly useless products. The good guys are being drowned out by the bad guys who only want to make a quick buck in a high selling market.

In such a situation, the responsibility rests with you to properly research the product and the company that is manufacturing it. Look for testimonials and reviews published on third party, neutral web sites. What sort of approvals does the product have? Are the ingredients checked for purity? What is the natural source for ingredients? What are the manufacturing standards that are being followed? How long has the company been in this business? These are all legitimate questions and usually you should be able to call up the company on a provided telephone number to have all your queries answered.

It does not matter what is the reason for your decision to take herbal supplements. It could be that you simply want an improvement in general health or you might be trying to combat some symptom that indicates the deficiency of some essential nutrient missing from your diet. What does matter is that you remember that when you go shopping for the supplement of your choice. An incorrectly chosen herbal supplement will plunge you into the group of people who think that all this "natural" business is so much humbug. A well chosen supplement on the other hand just might make you a convert and have you spreading the "natural" gospel to everyone you meet for the rest of your life.

NATURAL SKIN REMEDIES

Organic skin care refers to the use of natural skin care products or therapies. The ingredients of these natural products are grown organically in places that are rich in nutrients, unlike similar products that are purely manufactured using synthetic processes and ingredients.

Organic skin care makes use of several different types of plants, extracts, herbs, flowers, and natural oils. Organic skin care products are merely an extension of natural skin care therapies.

Organic skin care products are non-toxic and full of essential nutrients for the skin extracted from natural sources. These products nourish the skin and rejuvenate it gently. Some of the problems they can cure are dark circles, wrinkles, and pimples. The overall effect of organic skin care products is younger and healthier looking skin.

There are different organic skin care products available for the face and for other parts of the body. Since the structure of skin is different depending on the part body it is important to choose the appropriate product.

Apart from rejuvenating the skin, organic skin care products also have a soothing and healing effect on the body. Some of the ingredients are quite rich in soothing essences that have a calming effect. Organic skin care products can make you feel fresh in addition to nourishing your skin.

Newer products do not merely rely on plants and flowers. Some of them have already started using the special qualities of herbs and herbal extracts. Aloe vera, lavender, jojoba, olive oil, and rosemary extract are now regular ingredients in many organic skin care products.

Nourishment of the skin takes place through cleansing, moisturizing, and toning. Regular use of organic skin care products will ensure that your skin has no blemishes, pimples, or allergies.

These products also keep the skin soft and supple. Healthy skin will produce fewer wrinkles because of its firmness.

HERBAL ACNE REMEDIES

One of the more powerful forms of acne remedies is herbal. For people who are averse to taking strong acne drugs this is a very good option. The only problem with herbal remedies is that they are very slow acting and the results can take up to a month to become visible.

Even so, herbal acne home cures are a good side effort to whatever other treatments being used. The reason why herbal acne remedies take time is that these remedies depend on the body's capacity to metabolize fats and carbohydrates. Herbal remedies cure acne by encouraging the elimination of acne through the lymphatic system.

There is a class of herbs called "alternative herbs". These herbs are basically used for the purpose of cleansing body tissues. They are herbs that help the body with the detoxification process. However, they do not remove the toxins from the body through normal elimination pathways like lungs, kidneys, or colon.

While they are not so popular in western culture, herbal acne remedies have a long history of successfully treating acne problems and they are so harmless that you should at least give them one try. Moreover, since most herbal acne remedies work inside the body they do not interfere with conventional topical (applied externally) acne medications.

Alternative herbs are very mild acting so there is no discomfort in their use. However, since they are mild by nature they take a longer time and consistent use to show results. Despite this, the fact remains the results are better and longer lasting. What is more, these herbs usually have a beneficial affect on the rest of the body. They can even be used to treat chronic inflammatory conditions.

Some of the alternative herbs include burdock, cleavers, red clover, figwort, poke root, Echinacea, and blue flag.

Like most herbal remedies these herbal acne cures are also best when a combination of herbs is used. One frequently used and very popular combination is Echinacea, burdock, blue flag, and yellow dock. Just mix and prepare an infusion using hot water. Drink a cup about three times daily. If you wish to improve the flavor then please do no add sugar, instead, use honey.

A second combination is dandelion, sarsaparilla, and burdock. Mix them up when they are dry herbs. Prepare an infusion as before and have 3 cups a day.

A third decent combination for acne is lavender, yarrow, and elder flowers.

Besides these, herbal acne remedies are available for topical use.

Take the oil from a tea tree and apply it to the acne-affected area. This oil can be a bit strong so if you have sensitive skin just dilute it with water. Fresh cabbage juice makes another great topical herbal cure for acne. This is also a better choice for people with sensitive who cannot stand tea tree oil.

Calendula and chamomile can be used to make a very effective anti-inflammatory skin wash. Just prepare an infusion with these two as before but instead of drinking it let it cool. Store it in the fridge.

When required, dab it onto affected areas.

Minerals like potassium phosphate and magnesium phosphate are also good for the skin. Zinc aids in the prevention of scarring.

Vitamin C helps in healing acne lesions as well as acting as an anti-oxidant.

These are but a few cases of how herbal acne remedies can be of help.

NATURAL HERBAL RECIPE

It is very easy to make your own herbal medicines. In fact, since most herbal remedies are best consumed when they are at their freshest you even have the best of all choices: grown your own herbs and make your own fresh remedies.

However, it is important to have a thorough knowledge of the process of making your own remedies or even homegrown fresh herbs will go to waste.

Always keep in mind that unlike modern medicines herbal remedies are not a one-day affair. They take time to show their full effect because they work more gradually.

When preparing your own herbal remedies always use a non-metallic or enamel pot.

Infusions are mostly tea-like beverages that are made by combining fresh herbs and boiled water. The common method is steeping.

Typical ratios are about 1/2 or one ounce of herbs to one pint of boiled water. The mixture should be allowed to steep for at least 10 minutes. After that, you should strain the infusion into a cup.

Cold extracts make use of cold water instead of boiling water. The advantage is that unlike boiling some of the more volatile ingredients in herbs are not wasted in the extraction process. To prepare cold extracts, double the amount of herbal material and let it sit in cold water for about 12 hours then strain the mixture before drinking.

Decoction is a method of preparation that focuses on extracting mineral salts rather than vitamins. You should boil 1/2 ounce of herbs with one cup of water for 4-5 minutes. Steep the mixture for a couple of minutes before using it.

Juice from herbs should not be made in a blender. Just chop and crush the herbs to squeeze out the juice. Add some water to this concentrate and then squeeze some more, drink it immediately. Do not store juice extracted this way.

Powder can be made from grinding your herbs when they are dried. The powder can then be taken with water, milk, or soup.

Ointments can be prepared by adding olive oil to a previously prepared decoction and then putting it on simmer until the water has evaporated. Beeswax may be included to improve consistency.

Essence can be prepared by dissolving one ounce of essential herbal oil in a pint of alcohol.

Printed by Libri Plureos GmbH in Hamburg, Germany